COUPLES MASSAGE

A Couples Manual For Developing A Bond Through Massage

GATLIN ARES

Table of Contents

Introductory

In a couples massage, both people enjoy the therapeutic benefits of massage while sharing the same room with their therapist. One of the main goals of a couples massage is to establish a social setting where partners, friends, or family members can all enjoy the therapeutic benefits of massage together.

Couples massages are common at spas and massage treatment centers, and they may be a great way to relax and bond with your partner. Both customers can be assured of a synchronized and harmonic experience when the massage therapists harmonize their techniques and motions.

Couples massage not only helps you relax and unwind, but it also gives you a chance to spend quality time with your partner in a peaceful and relaxing environment. It can be a chance for couples to spend quality time together, a spa day for families, or an opportunity for friends to bond over shared interests.

Each partner in a couples massage may have their own unique experience, so the massage can be as relaxing or therapeutic as the couple desires.

CHAPTER ONE
Various Methods For Couples Massage

Couples massages can be tailored to suit the preferences and needs of those who partake. During a massage for two, the therapist may use a wide variety of techniques and styles. Couples massage often takes the following forms:

• Long, smooth strokes, circular motions, and kneading make up Swedish massage, a calming and relaxing technique. Improving circulation and promoting relaxation are its two main functions.

• Deep Tissue Massage: This method focuses on the underlying layers of muscle and connective tissue. Regularly used to alleviate persistent aches and pains as well as acute muscular tension, it might be even more vigorous than Swedish massage.

• Hot stone massage: this technique involves placing heated stones on certain areas of the body in order to alleviate muscle tension and stress. To further enhance the therapeutic and calming effects of the massage, the therapist may also choose to use the stones for other purposes.

• Aromatherapy Massage: Adding aromatic essential oils to a massage can greatly improve its therapeutic effects. A variety of oils have different effects that can help you relax, feel better emotionally, or ease muscle tension.

• Compression, rhythmic motions, and aided flexibility are the main components of a Thai massage. Participants usually wear loose, comfortable clothing and do it on a floor mat.

• Muscle injuries and strains are the main areas of concentration when it comes to sports massage. Additional treatment procedures may be employed alongside deep tissue techniques and stretching.

• Originally from Japan, shiatsu massage focuses on releasing tension in certain areas of the body to improve energy flow. It usually involves stretching and joint mobilization, and the recipient isn't even supposed to be fully dressed the whole time.

• Ayurveda is an old Indian medical system; it includes a couples massage. Depending on the patient's dosha (consstitution), an Ayurvedic massage may use heated oils and other techniques.

When scheduling a couple's massage, be sure to let the therapists know your priorities, any sore spots, and the pressure you'd like applied. This method improves the atmosphere while making sure the massage is personalized to meet the needs of the client.

Setting Apart From One-On-One Massage

The primary difference between a couple's massage and an individual's massage is the setting and the number of people receiving the service. Listed below are a number of key distinctions:

• Two people can get a massage at the same time in the same room if they book a couples massage.

• Everyone in the group, whether it's a spouse, coworker, or family member, can enjoy the therapeutic effects of massage.

• In contrast, a single receiver is the focus of a solo massage.

• Depending on the couple's preferences and comfort level, they might choose to have their massage in the same room or separate ones. The client usually reclines in a quiet room while receiving a one-on-one massage.

• Synchronized Massage: When massaging a couple, the therapists may find it enjoyable to match their strokes in time with one another. The coordination adds a special touch to the session and makes the shared experience even better.

• Many people see couples massages as a way to bond with one another while also providing a shared experience of relaxation. A chance to relax and enjoy a peaceful time together, it's perfect for families, friends, and couples. Personal massages, on the other hand, are more customized to meet the specific needs of each client in terms of relaxation and therapeutic effects.

• Both couples and individuals can have their massages customized to meet their own preferences and needs. Nevertheless, when massaging a couple, therapists may need to take into account each client's unique tastes and adjust the session appropriately.

• Both couples massages and solo massages rely heavily on conversation; but, when two people are getting massaged together, there may be an extra layer of conversation. Clients have the option of engaging in conversation, enjoying the massage in privacy, or communicating their preferences directly to the therapists.

• The romantic or intimate atmosphere often linked with couples massages makes them popular among couples who want to spend quality time together.

• Candlelight, soothing music, or other one-of-a-kind ambient features can all contribute to a more romantic atmosphere.

Couples massage differs from individual massages in that it is performed in a more intimate setting and the couples have more pleasure throughout the session, even though the basic principles of massage treatment are the same.

Both types of massage are tailored to the specific needs of each client and can help with a variety of issues, including stress reduction, relaxation, and therapeutic effects.

What Communication Is Crucial

Massage therapy relies heavily on open communication, whether the client is a couple or an individual. There are a number of reasons why good communication is crucial during a massage:

1. Modification for the One-on-One Massage:

• The massage therapist can tailor the session to your exact needs if you let them know your preferences, such as the amount of pressure you want applied, which regions you want worked on, and if you're in any pain or discomfort.

• To make sure that a couples massage is enjoyable for both people, it's a good idea for them to let the masseuse know what they want.

2. Ease and Safety:

• Before beginning the massage, please inform the therapist of any current or past health issues, injuries, or worries that could compromise your safety or well-being.

• If you notice any pain throughout the massage, whether it's from the lighting, the temperature of the room, or the pressure level, please let the therapist know so that they may make the necessary adjustments to ensure your comfort.

3. Notes Taken During the Massage:

• Feedback given at various points of the massage is helpful. The therapist can maximize your experience by making real-time adjustments if the pressure is too intense or not profound enough.

• To make sure both partners are comfortable and happy during the massage, they can communicate with one other and the therapists.

4. Comfort on a Mental and Emotional Level:

• Massage therapy offers emotional and psychological advantages. By opening up about how you're feeling, the therapist can create a supportive and calming environment.

• It's common for couples to talk about their massages while they're getting them, which can help them relax and bond with one another.

5. The Informed Parties' Consent:

• The therapist will usually go over the massage's objectives and the specific methods that will be used before the session even begins. Open and honest dialogue about the suggested method can help get everyone on the same page and share relevant information.

6. The modification of approaches:

• A wide variety of techniques are taught to massage therapists during their training. You can help your therapist better meet your needs by letting them know if you have a preference for a certain approach.

7. Practical and Factors That Promote Relaxation:

• It is possible to achieve a state of deep relaxation during a massage if the therapist and client are able to communicate effectively. Improving one's body awareness and effectively expressing one's needs enhances the therapeutic benefits of massage by creating an atmosphere of mindfulness during the session.

• Honest and honest communication is a two-way street, so keep that in mind. To ensure a pleasant and effective encounter, it is essential for both the therapist and the client to actively participate.

For a couples massage to be an enjoyable and memorable experience for both partners, it is essential that they be able to communicate well with the therapists.

CHAPTER TWO
Assembling The Massage Table

If you want to get the most out of your massage, it's a good idea to do some before preparation. Whatever kind of massage you're planning—a couple's or an individual session—the following tips will help you get ready:

1. Having Conversations with the Massage Therapist:

• You should let the massage therapist know about any injuries, health issues, or problem regions in your body either during the first consultation or before the session starts if you have any.

• Describe your ideal massage pressure, whether you want to use oil or lotion, and the exact techniques that bring you the most relief.

2. When it comes to personal hygiene:

• Take a bath or shower to make sure you're clean and rejuvenated before the massage.

• Keep light perfumes and colognes at arm's length; they might interfere with the massage.

3. What to Wear:

• Wear comfortable clothing if you plan on visiting a massage therapy clinic or retreat. A robe or some disposable underwear might be provided to you if you need them.

• Dress comfortably in casual, loose-fitting garments since some massage styles, like Thai massage, may necessitate going naked.

4. Considering the time:

• To promote an environment of relaxation and leisure, it is recommended that you arrive promptly for your appointment.

• Make sure to show up simultaneously with your companion if it's a couples massage.

5. Hydration to an adequate level:

• Drink water before and after getting a massage to keep yourself hydrated. A combination of massage and adequate hydration can help flush toxins out of the muscles.

6. Practicing relaxation and meditation:

• Take some time to relax and relax before the massage. To improve the experience overall and soothe the nervous system, try some deep breathing exercises or meditation.

• Turning off or putting your phone in silent mode can help reduce distractions.

7. Jewelry and accessories:

• To avoid interfering with the therapist's job, take off any jewelry or other items before the massage.

• Keep all valuable possessions in the lockers or another specified areas provided by the institution.

8. Expectations Regarding Couples Massage:

• It is recommended that you and your partner talk about your desires and expectations before getting a couples massage. All of your special requests, such whether you prefer a communal or private room, as well as any extras you might want, like music or aromatherapy, will be considered.

9. Strategies to Follow Before a Massage:

• Get back to organizing your schedule after the massage. After that, it's always a good idea to plan some downtime instead of jumping back into a busy schedule right once.

10. As an extra favor:

• If the spa's policies don't state otherwise, please bring cash or a credit card to cover the gratuity.

• Having open lines of communication with your massage

therapist and your partner is crucial when getting a couples massage.

The therapist's ability to tailor the massage to your needs is directly proportional to how well they understand your tastes and any issues you may have. The advantages of your massage will be greatly enhanced if you follow these steps.

Essential Methods Of Massage

It all depends on the goals of the massage as well as the recipient's preferences; different sections of the body can benefit from different massage techniques. Fundamental massage techniques commonly used by massage therapists include:

1. How effleurage works:

• To get the muscles ready for a deeper massage, a therapist will use long, wide strokes to warm them up.

• Light to moderate pressure applied with the fingertips as they glide over the skin is the key to this technique.

2. "Petrisage" means:

• Movements like rolling, pushing, and squeezing the muscles are all part of kneading and compression exercises. To improve blood flow and alleviate stress, petrissage is a common technique.

3. The force due to friction:

• To create heat and break down adhesions in muscles, move the palms, fingers, or thumbs in a circular or transverse motion. Friction is a useful way to reduce stress in specific areas.

4. The term "tapotement" means:

• The use of hacking, pounding, cupping, and other rhythmic hitting and percussive motions. One rejuvenating method is tapotement, which helps with both stress release and increased blood flow.

5. Vibration:

• The user uses their hands or fingers to make quick, accurate shaking or swaying movements.

• A lot of people use vibration to help with muscle pain and relaxation.

6. The procedure for compressing:

• Regularly pressing down on a specific spot with the palms of the hands or fingers. Compression is a great tool for relieving muscle tension and releasing trigger points.

7. The elevation:

• You may increase your flexibility and range of motion by gently stretching your muscles and joints. In many massage styles, including Thai massage, stretching is an integral part of the treatment.

8. Engaging Joints:

• In order to increase range of motion and decrease stiffness in the joints, the massage therapist will use passive joint movements. It is common practice to use this in conjunction with other massage techniques.

9. Myofascial Tissue Release:

• The fascia, a kind of connective tissue, can be relaxed and energy flow increased by applying gentle, sustained pressure. Myofascial release is frequently used to alleviate persistent pain and stress.

10. Therapy at the point of trigger:

• Muscle trigger points can be used to relieve pain and tension by applying sustained pressure to specific areas.

Areas of concern are often targeted using this strategy.

11. Friction between Fibers:

• Scar tissue and adhesions can be eradicated by applying particular pressure along the fibers of the muscle. There is hope that cross-fiber friction can help in injury treatment and tissue regeneration.

There are several elements that should be considered while choosing massage techniques. These include the client's preferences, the goals of the massage, and any specific health issues that need to be addressed.

In addition, skilled massage therapists may often combine several approaches to create a unique and effective treatment plan for each client.

If you have any special requests, concerns, or are experiencing pain during your massage, please do not hesitate to let your therapist know.

CHAPTER THREE
Techniques For Making A Connection

By using specific approaches, the general rapport between participants in common experiences like couples massages can be enhanced, which in turn fosters a sense of connectedness. Here are a few ways to encourage bonding:

1. Taking a Deep Breath:

• Start the workout by breathing deliberately together for a short length of time. Breathe in and out slowly, matching the rhythm of your partner's breath. Not only does this help you unwind, but it also sets a rhythm that everyone can enjoy.

2. Being Present:

• Inspire each other to stay fully present in the here and now. Pay close attention to your feelings, sensations, and the sounds that surround you as the massage progresses. Being fully present in the moment of shared experience deepens the bond.

3. Coordinating Physical Movements:

• Synchronized movements should be incorporated into a couple's massage. Encourage the two people to move or alter positions at the same time, as long as they are comfortable with it, to create a balanced and linked flow.

4. Communicating Through Body Language:

• Show your affection by using soft touches or non-verbal cues. Just a little squeeze or a comforting pat on the shoulder will do the trick. Through the use of nonverbal cues, a stronger sense of connection can be established.

5. Establishment of Mutual Goals:

• It's a good idea to have a chat and make plans to meet before the massage. This may include goals like relieving stress or just spending quality time together. A cohesive focus can be achieved by coordinating intentions.

6. Show Your Gratitude:

• Take a moment before or after the massage to express your gratitude to the other person. Show your appreciation for each other and the experience. Expressing gratitude strengthens the emotional relationship and amplifies good emotions.

7.   Interactions   Occurring Throughout the Massage:

• Feel free to talk to each other and the massage therapists about your session if you're comfortable doing so. You can enhance the communal nature of the experience by discussing the sensations or preferences in real-time.

8. Ways to Relax Your Muscles:

• Use strategies for joint relaxation that both people can actively participate in. Gentle joint movements, synchronized breathing exercises, or companion stretches may all fall within this category.

9. Regular Practices:

• Incorporate group practices or ceremonies into the activity. This could entail a specific order of events leading up to or after the massage, like a quiet chat between the couple or a simple hand gesture.

10. Reflecting on the Massage Aftereffects:

• Take a moment to reflect as a group after the massage. Give some background on how you felt and what you enjoyed best about the experience. Sharing thoughts and feelings strengthens relationships and creates positive memories.

11. Create a Friendly Atmosphere:

• A massaging setting that encourages connection must be established. Aromatherapy, soothing music, or lighting alterations could all help with this. Remember that being sensitive to one another's comfort levels and preferences is essential for creating an engaging and pleasant setting, which enhances the whole experience.

These strategies can be adjusted to create a better sense of connection by taking into account the unique dynamics of the participants.

Creating Unique Massage Experiences For Each Other

Personalizing massages for a loved one can be a relaxing and intimate way to spend quality time together in a romantic setting. Here is some guidance to help you make your partner's massages more special:

1.   Mastering   Effective Communication:

• Before you start talking, think about each other's preferences, potential grounds of dispute, and how intense you want the conversation to be. For a massage to be both relaxing and tailored to each client's needs, clear and open communication is essential.

2. Methodology Selection:

• I recommend tailoring your massage to your partner's tastes by incorporating a range of techniques. Some people may feel more comfortable with gentler approaches and fewer strokes, while others may benefit from deeper pressure.

3. Zero in on problem areas:

• Ask your friend if there's anywhere on their body that can use some extra TLC. This could be related to a region plagued with constant discomfort or a particular set of muscles marked by ongoing stress.

4. Using Oils and Lotions:

• Ask your partner if they like oil or lotion; it's not a personal question. Some people may prefer scented oils to unscented ones when it comes to aromatherapy. Check your partner's skin type to be sure the product you've chosen is suitable.

5. Environment and thermostat:

• The current weather and the surrounding conditions should be considered. Make sure the room is warm enough, and then adjust the lights and music to create a soothing atmosphere.

6. Incorporate Personal Touches:

• Make the massage more unique by adding features that are specific to the client. Things like playing music with emotional value, adding a favorite scent, or using a particular massage oil can fall under this category.

7. Evaluate and Try Out Methods:

• Feel free to experiment with different massage methods until you find one that your spouse enjoys the most. Gently stretching, kneading, or even a variety of strokes could be part of this.

Ask for comments as you go forward with the massage. Look over your travel partner to make sure they're relaxed and having fun. This allows for the implementation of changes in real-time.

8. Set the Stage for Relaxation:

• To create a peaceful atmosphere, pay attention to the little things. Put on some calming music, turn down the lights, and make sure nobody is around to disturb you.

9. A Gentle Caress:

• Listen to your gut and watch your partner's body language. Adjust your touch based on their responses for a more pleasurable and relaxing encounter.

10. Post-Massage Care:

• Give your massage partner some space to relax afterward. To make the most of your post-massage relaxation, consider providing a warm towel or a calming drink.

• When massaging each other to perfection, it is essential to be fully present and communicate with each other.

Being open and receptive to your partner's cues and feedback will improve the experience and make it more enjoyable for everyone involved, since everyone has different inclinations and sensitivity levels.

CHAPTER FOUR
An Aromatherapy Approach

By invigorating the sense of smell and promoting relaxation, aromatherapy can enhance the whole massage experience. For those who want to enjoy their massages in a couple's setting, here are a few ways to incorporate aromatherapy:

1. Choose Calming Aromatic Tone Sets:

• Pick out some essential oils that are known to be soothing. Standard choices include bergamot, lavender, chamomile, and ylang-ylang. Reportedly, these aromas might help you relax.

2. Dilution of Essential Oil:

• Essential oils should be diluted in a carrier oil before being applied topically. Carrier oils are commonly found in jojoba, sweet almond, and coconut oils. That way, you can be sure that the essential oils you apply to your skin will do their job without harm.

3. Setting the Scene for Relaxation:

• To create the ideal aroma for a massage, use an essential oil diffuser. On the other hand, you may dab a tissue or cloth with a few drops of the essential oil and scatter it throughout the room.

4. Meet the Unique Needs of Each Customer:

• Have a discussion with your partner about your preferred scents. Some people may have a strong inclination for certain aromas that they find very relaxing or enjoyable. Making aromatherapy more unique by tailoring it to each individual's needs.

5. Blending Scents for an Unconventional Pleasure:

• Experimenting with different combinations of essential oils to create an unmatched aroma is an option. For a stimulating and calming combination, try combining lavender with a citrus scent, for instance.

6. Apply diluted oil to the skin:

• Try dabbing some essential oils into your partner's skin if they like skin-to-skin contact. The temples, wrists, and neck should be your primary foci. To avoid skin irritation, make sure to choose a dilution ratio that is safe.

7. Oils should be heated:

• The massage oils are best used after they have been warmed. To achieve this, just place the oil in a basin of warm water and let it soak for a few minutes. Aromatherapy with warm oils can stimulate the senses.

8. Use Candles for Aromatherapy:

• You can increase the aesthetic and fragrant aspects of the massage area by opting for candles that are infused with essential oils. Put the candles somewhere safe, far from where you'll be massaging.

9. Supply of Neck Wraps for Aromatherapy:

• Scented rice or herbs can be used to make aromatherapy neck wraps or eye pillows. To make the massage more relaxing, you might put them over your eyelids or around your neck.

10. Addressing Sensitivities:

• Find out if your partner has any allergies or sensitivities before you use aromatherapy. This guarantees that the selected aromas are pleasant and non-irritating.

11. Aromatherapy for Follow-Up Massages:

• Even after the massage is over, you can continue to benefit from aromatherapy. To ensure that your relaxation lasts, consider providing scented towels or an aromatic bath.

Always check with your partner to see if they have any smell preferences or sensitivities; after all, everyone has different tastes. When combined with massage, aromatherapy creates a lovely multi-sensory experience that is sure to soothe both people.

Dealing With Common Challenges

Massages have the potential to bring about intense feelings of pleasure and relaxation, but they do have some common challenges. Some possible solutions to these problems are as follows:

• If you are experiencing pain or discomfort during your massage, it is important to communicate openly with your therapist about how bad it is. Never be afraid to voice your issue if the pressure gets too much. In order to cater to your individual preferences, a skilled massage therapist will adjust their method.

• If you are sensitive to ticklishness, the best course of action is to let your massage therapist know before your session begins. Applying more firm pressure or avoiding too sensitive areas are two potential adjustments. If you're experiencing ticklish feelings, try focusing on deep breathing exercises.

• Resolving an Adverse Dialogue: If you would want a calm and relaxing experience, please let the massage therapist know before the session begins. The vast majority of medical professionals will respect your need for privacy.

• Resolving the Feeling of Cold or Heat: Not everyone has the same ideal temperature for the massage room. Telling the therapist how comfortable you are will allow them to adjust the room's temperature or provide additional blankets or fans.

• Resolving Embarrassment or Self-Consciousness: In the first few minutes of getting a massage, you may feel a little self-conscious. Remember that massage therapists are experts in their field whose main goal is to make sure you have a good time. If you have any specific worries, let the therapist know before your session.

• Stop tensing up and start focusing on your breathing if you're having trouble relaxing. If you would like the therapist to focus on particular areas where you are feeling particularly anxious or stressed, please let them know.

• Fixing Uncomfortable placement: Tell your therapist if the bolstering or placement is making you feel uncomfortable. Feel safe and at ease knowing that adjustments can be made to meet your needs.

• Pain After a Massage: How to Get Rid of It: Muscle aches and pains are common, especially after a deep tissue massage. Stay well hydrated, use hot or cold compresses as needed, and let the therapist know if the pressure is too much.

• Problem Solved: Talk to your massage therapist if you feel like there's a lot of oil or lotion left over after the session. You have the option to ask for less oil or ask for cloths to soak up any excess.

• Resolving Unexpected Emotional Reactions: Massage can occasionally trigger emotional reactions. When overwhelming emotions strike, it's important to acknowledge and express them. The connection between the body and the intellect includes it intrinsically.

• If you have any allergies or sensitivities to certain oils or lotions, it's best to let the massage therapist know before the session begins.

If we are to successfully face these problems, we must maintain an open channel of communication. By vocalizing your preferences, worries, or unexpected reactions to the massage therapist, you may help create an atmosphere that is comfortable and pleasant for everyone involved.

CHAPTER FIVE
Tips For A Relaxing Couples Massage

Sharing a massage as a couple can be a romantic and relaxing way to unwind. To ensure a pleasant couple's massage, follow these steps:

• Prefer an Appropriate Setting: Set aside a peaceful and cozy spot to enjoy the massage. It could happen in a retreat, in the privacy of one's own home, or some other place famous for its serene atmosphere.

• Make a pact to discuss each other's massage preferences before the session begins. Be sure to address any health issues or sensitivities, the amount of pressure, and the regions of concentration.

• Create the Mood: Low-key lighting, soothing music, and maybe some aromatic candles or essential oils can all contribute to a relaxing ambiance. A sense of calm should permeate the space.

• Start the Massage: A gentle warm-up should be performed before the massage begins. Build up your muscles for more strenuous activity by gradually increasing the pressure and using broad strokes.

• If you and your friend feel comfortable doing so, try to coordinate your movements. If you and your partner can move in sync or switch positions, this could lead to a relaxing encounter.

• Be respectful of one another's boundaries and personal space. As the massage progresses, make sure your partner is comfortable with the pressure and techniques used.

• Do not be shy about trying out different massage techniques; this is an important part of the learning process. Find the technique that works best for you by experimenting with different combinations of kneading, gentle stretches, and strokes.

• Choose High-Quality Massage Oils and Moisturizers and Use Them. Think about aromatherapy if you and your partner enjoy scented products; just be careful not to trigger anyone's allergies or sensitivities.

• Attention to Temperature: Keep the chamber at a temperature that is comfortable. To cater to different tastes, feel free to provide extra towels or blankets.

• Keep the lines of communication open as much as possible during the massage. If your spouse experiences any unexpected discomfort or excitement, be sure to inform them. It makes the shared experience better.

• To ensure that both you and your companion get the most out of your massages, try switching roles every so often. Both people involved should care about the outcome because it is a group effort.

• After your massage, take some time to unwind and rest. Provide a comfortable spot for your pet to rest and drink water or a soothing drink to keep them hydrated.

• Respond to the message by sharing your thoughts and opinions with the other recipients. Evaluate the success of the project and decide if any changes are required for the future.

• Proposal for After the Massage: Plan some downtime or quality time together after the massage.

Indulging in a long, leisurely activity, like taking a bath, having a romantic meal, or simply cuddling, can greatly enhance the overall experience.

Keep in mind that creating a peaceful and supportive atmosphere, as well as communicating and respecting one another, are essential for a successful couples massage.

Take pleasure in the shared moments of connection and relaxation by tailoring the experience to the interests of both companions.

Help From Industry Professionals And Ongoing Training

To maintain a successful and fulfilling career, massage therapists must seek professional advice and participate in continuous education. Massage therapists can further their education and access professional help in the following ways:

• Supervision and Mentorship: Enroll in programs that pair you with more seasoned healthcare professionals or massage therapists to learn the ropes. Advice, criticism, and the sharing of information can all be more easily provided in this way.

• You should consider becoming a member of an organization or association that focuses on professional massage treatment. These groups often supply members with resources, introduce them to one another, and grant them admission to conferences and seminars.

• Regularly Participate in Workshops and Seminars: Keep abreast of the latest developments in your field by attending relevant workshops and seminars. You may learn a lot from the experts in your field at these events.

It is recommended to obtain advanced qualifications and

specializations in specific massage modalities or methods. In addition to enhancing one's skill set, this action demonstrates a commitment to continuous professional development.

• Collaborating with coworkers and peers: Exchanging information and insights in this way. Significant insights and practical guidance may be uncovered through peer learning.

• Clinical Conferences: Take part in clinical conferences discussing topics related to therapy, wellness, and healthcare. Renowned speakers and hands-on workshops at these conferences help professionals learn more about a variety of topics.

• Journals and Literature: By perusing scholarly publications, books, and online resources relating to massage therapy and allied health. One way to help put evidence-based practice into action is to keep up with the latest research and industry literature.

• Look at schools that provide advanced massage therapy methods as a possible place to further your education. Comprehensive programs to improve one's skill set are often offered by these schools.

• Individual Plans for Professional growth: Make a detailed plan for your own professional growth that specifies your goals in terms of education, credentials, and skill enhancement. In order to keep track of how things are going, you should review and update this plan often.

• Consider joining a therapist support group or forum if you are looking for advice, want to make relationships with other professionals, and want to share your story. You can find support and camaraderie through groups both online and in your local area.

• Consultation with Other Medical Experts: Encourage interdisciplinary training through teamwork with other medical experts, such as chiropractors and physical therapists. The therapist's knowledge of alternative medicine may grow as a result.

• Core Competencies: If you want to learn more than just massage methods, you should sign up for classes on corporate ethics, effective communication, and management.

Maintaining one's physical and emotional well-being should be a top priority, thus make self-care a priority. This could include doing things like getting regular exercise, being attentive, and finding ways to balance your personal and professional lives.

Maintaining and improving one's skills, as well as staying current on industry advancements and best practices, are both made possible through continuing education.

It shows that you care about your clients and always act in a professional manner. In addition, getting help from a professional, whether it's for career advice or mental health issues, is crucial if you want your massage therapy job to thrive and last.

Summary

Massage therapy is an enjoyable and complex field that uses many different approaches to improve people's physical and mental well-being.

When massage therapists and clients alike are well-versed in the many techniques used in the field, understand the value of open and honest communication, and are able to tailor treatments to each client's unique needs, everyone benefits.

If you want to be successful and happy as a massage therapist, you need to commit to ongoing professional development, find a mentor, and keep up with industry developments.

Guaranteeing superior care to clients is the goal of therapists who stay current on recent research and methodologies and use sophisticated techniques.

Making the recipient more aware of their breath during the massage, encouraging open dialogue with the therapist, and creating a relaxing atmosphere are all ways to improve the quality of the massage and its therapeutic effects.

Personalizing the massage to each person's tastes and needs is the key to making it an unforgettable experience, whether it's for two or one.

Keep in mind that massage therapy is more than just working on the muscles; it takes a more holistic view by considering the mind-body connection. Massage has many uses, including the alleviation of stress and anxiety as well as the treatment of some musculoskeletal disorders.

If massage therapy is to continue evolving into a more effective and widely used therapeutic modality, it is imperative that both therapists and patients take an active role in shaping its future.

Whether giving or receiving a massage, the goal is the same: to improve health and happiness.

THE END